ACE Group Fitness Specialty Book

Step
Training

by Sabra Bonelli, M.S.

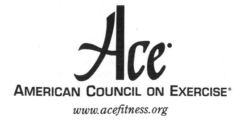

AMERICAN COUNCIL ON EXERCISE®
www.acefitness.org

Library of Congress Catalog Card Number: 00-104273

First edition
ISBN 1-890720-02-X
Copyright © 2000 American Council on Exercise® (ACE®)
Printed in the United States of America.

A B C D E F

Distributed by:
American Council on Exercise
P. O. Box 910449
San Diego, CA 92191-0449
(858) 535-8227
(858) 535-1778 (FAX)
www.acefitness.org

Managing Editor: Daniel Green
Design: Karen McGuire
Production: Glenn Valentine
Manager of Publications: Christine Ekeroth
Associate Editor: Joy Keller
Index: Bonny McLaughlin
Model: Betsy Wellman

Acknowledgements:
Thanks to the entire American Council on Exercise staff for their support and guidance through the process of creating this manual.

NOTICE
The fitness industry is ever-changing. As new research and clinical experience broaden our knowledge, changes in programming and standards are required. The authors and the publisher of this work have checked with sources believed to be reliable in their efforts to provide information that is complete and generally in accord with the standards accepted at the time of publication. However, in view of the possibility of human error or changes in industry standards, neither the authors nor the publisher nor any other party who has been involved in the preparation or publication of this work warrants that the information contained herein is in every respect accurate or complete, and they are not responsible for any errors or omissions or the results obtained from the use of such information. Readers are encouraged to confirm the information contained herein with other sources.

REVIEWERS

Lorna Francis, Ph.D., previously a physical education professor at San Diego State University, is an internationally recognized speaker and the author of several fitness books. An ACE-certified instructor, Dr. Francis is an emeritus member of ACE's board of directors and was co-recipient of the 1989 IDEA Lifetime Achievement award.

Denise Tucker is a Reebok Master Trainer and national trainer for Resist-A-Ball. She contributed to several Reebok University Specialty Programs and was a development team member for Reebok Flexible Strength. Active as an ACE- and NASM-certified Personal Trainer, Tucker spent 10 years as an assistant strength and conditioning coach for a New England high school. She is an ACE spokesperson and has contributed articles to fitness publications, including *Fitness, Shape,* and *American Fitness.*

TABLE OF
CONTENTS

INTRODUCTION

T he American Council on Exercise
(ACE) is pleased to include
Step Training as a Group Fitness
Specialty Book. As the industry con-
tinues to expand, evolve, and redefine itself, step training
has emerged as a viable component of fitness. Guidelines
and criteria have been established so that this exercise
modality can be practiced both safely and effectively. The
intent of this book is to educate and give guidance to fitness professionals that wish to teach step training. As with
all areas of fitness, education is a continual process. ACE
recognizes this is a broad subject requiring serious study
and we encourage you to use the References and
Suggested Reading to further your knowledge.

Chapter One

Introduction to Step Training

Since the first stirrings of the physical fitness craze in the early 1970s, no development has revolutionized the fitness industry more than step aerobics, which was introduced in the late 1980s. Also called bench aerobics, step/bench training, and aerobic stepping, step training is a relatively low-impact exercise program that utilizes a platform ranging from 4 to 12 inches in height. Participants step up and down performing a variety of movement skills and sequences to music, utilizing large muscle groups to tax the cardiovascular, respiratory, and muscular systems. Since its inception, the popularity of step training as a means of achieving and/or maintaining aerobic fitness has continually skyrocketed, with recent estimates reporting that more than 11 million people in over 40 countries participate in step training regularly (Scharff-Olson & Williford, 1998).

History

The physiological response to stepping up and down off a bench has been known for decades. Exercise physiologists in the early 20th century developed fitness tests based on the heart-rate response to repetitive stepping, such as the Harvard Step Test. Clinicians more recently have employed step tests for the purpose of assessing functional capacity and/or detecting cardiovascular disease. Further step-test protocols have been developed and validated in major universities for estimating physical work capacity and aerobic fitness. For example, Fred Kasch, Ph.D., of San Diego State University developed the 3-Minute Step Test, which is currently used by YMCAs for mass testing of participants.

The most common medical use of stepping has been in rehabilitation. For cardiac rehabilitation purposes bench stepping is a highly controlled way of increasing the metabolic cost of exercise to a level slightly higher than walking. This is particularly useful for cardiac patients, as step training works the muscles used to climb stairs, providing a great functional application. Stepping is also used in sports medicine rehabilitation, most specifically as a standard form of knee rehabilitation exercise. Stepping emphasizes conditioning the quadriceps muscles, which are important for knee stability, provides low injury potential to the recovering knee due to its low-impact nature, and is an ideal progressive exercise for knee rehabilitation because of its adjustability and control. It was the use of stepping in knee rehabilitation that ultimately led to a revolution in the fitness industry.

In 1989, Reebok University (an exercise research and educational group supported by Reebok International) helped launch the use of step training in group exercise settings by combining bench stepping with aerobic dance techniques. Reebok trainers traveled the globe presenting step programming to fitness professionals and consumers, while researchers began the process of establishing step training as a safe and effective aerobic training modality.

Growth

Aerobic dance exercise has long been one of the most popular exercise modes among adult women in America, with an estimated 23 million participants at the peak of its popularity in the mid-1980s (Koszuta, 1986). Step exercise evolved primarily out of a need for another type of challenging, interesting, and effective cardiovascular activity. Despite the advent of complex choreography and power step training, which utilizes hops and jumps to increase intensity, it is the relatively low-impact nature of the exercise that has largely contributed to the popularity of step training.

By the early 1990s step training was in use virtually worldwide. Designed to be a predominantly low-impact, high-intensity athletic activity, it attracted men and women of all ages. People who had otherwise avoided group exercise aerobics classes due to the choreographed, "dancey" movements were initially attracted to step training due to the nonintimidating, basic movements. The generally accepted terminology and predictable, defined environment (each participant works in the space defined by the platform) aided in the growing success of step training.

An additional dimension to the growth of step exercise is its versatility. Within a few years of its launch as a primarily simple and athletic low-impact aerobic class format, a variety of alternative class modalities utilizing the step were developed and introduced. These include classes such as interval training, circuit training, muscular conditioning, combination classes, which combine aerobic stepping with high- and/or low-impact aerobics, step classes that involve active use of more than one platform, classes based on skill level, and classes known as power step, which utilize high-impact moves. Such versatility only increased the popularity of step training and broadened its appeal. By the late 1990s, step training had become a highly commercialized global phenomenon, considered an essential part of any complete group exercise class schedule.

Benefits

Cardiorespiratory Training

Step training is a moderate-to-high intensity aerobic activity that effectively challenges the cardiorespiratory system. The overall energy cost depends on the type of step movements used during a class. Research at Adelphi University (Calarco et al., 1991) was done using a 6-inch platform. Energy cost in METS varied from 7.5 for a basic step, to 9.1 for a lunge. (One MET, or metabolic equivalent, is the amount of oxygen required per minute under resting conditions, or 3.5 milliliters of oxygen per kilogram of body weight per minute.) In a study at San Diego State University, testing on an 8-inch platform revealed that a class utilizing non-propulsive step patterns and arm movements averaged 7.7 METS, a value comparable to traditional hi/lo aerobic dance (Francis et al., 1992). Woodby-Brown et al. (1993) studied the oxygen cost of aerobic dance bench stepping and found that step has oxygen requirements similar to other forms of aerobic dance, providing appropriate intensity challenges for improving aerobic fitness. Stanforth et al. (1993) and Williford et al. (1995) also found step training to significantly improve aerobic capacity.

Weight Management

Several studies have evaluated the energy expenditure of step training to determine its usefulness in weight control. Keeping in mind that dietary control and frequency of training affect weight loss and maintenance efforts, researchers have examined step training solely in terms of caloric costs. Scharff-Olson et al. (1991) studied step exercise and energy expenditure (Figure 1). It was determined that for participants desiring weight or fat loss, step exercise must be performed for longer than 20 minutes to expend the minimum 200 kcal/session recommended by ACSM (1995).

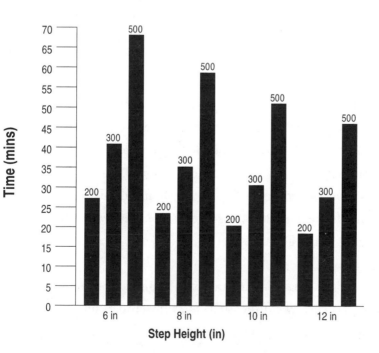

Figure 1
The number of minutes necessary to expend 200, 300, and 500 kcal at various step heights.
(Reprinted with permission from Scharff-Olson et al., 1991.)

Preliminary studies revealed the energy cost of step training to be between 6 and 11 METS, resulting in an energy expenditure of 6 to 11 kcal/min (La Forge, 1991). Studies have shown that energy cost increases steadily as step height is raised from 4 to 12 inches (Francis, 1993). This is true with the use of both basic step patterns (Stanforth et al., 1993) and choreographed routines (Rupp et al., 1992; Scharff-Olson et al., 1991). Studies on the use of plyometric or power moves (e.g., lunges) have shown such step patterns to increase the energy requirements of step training up to 17% above the basic step across a variety of step heights from 6 to 12 inches (Scharff-Olson & Williford, 1996). A study of power-step movements by Francis et al. (1992) examined the MET cost of stepping at 120 beats per minute (bpm) on an 8-inch platform. Results revealed a legs-only basic step routine yielded 6.9 METS and a basic step routine with arm movements yielded 7.7 METS. A power routine yielded 10.6 METS, increasing the energy cost of stepping by almost 54% over the legs-only routine.

Additionally, body weight plays a large role in the amount of calories expended during step training. Combining all factors, including step height, step rate, body weight, and step patterns, makes it difficult to determine the actual number of calories expended in a step-training session (Scharff-Olson & Williford, 1998). Table 1 shows the number of minutes of basic step exercise needed to burn 300 kcals on different platform heights at different body weights.

Adaptability

One of the greatest benefits of step training is its appropriateness for a variety of fitness levels. Many studies have demonstrated that step is easily modified according to fitness needs by

Table 1
Time (minutes) to burn 300 kcals for various body weights and platform heights

Weight		Platform Height		
(pounds)	(kg)	6 inches	8 inches	10 inches
120	54	40	38	36
130	59	36	34	32
140	63	34	32	30
150	68	32	30	28
160	72	30	28	26
170	77	28	26	24
180	81	26	24	22

The time necessary to expend 300 kcal ranges substantially depending on body weight and step height. For health purposes, a 50% reduction in any time value will yield the minutes of step training needed to meet the 150 kcal criterion.

adjusting step height (Scharff-Olson et al., 1991; Stanforth et al., 1993). Participants at a beginning level can use the 4-inch step height. As they become familiar with stepping techniques and their fitness level improves, the height of the platform can be increased, demanding greater intensity. If step height adjustments are not appropriate, you can also increase step cadence to achieve greater intensity (Goss et al., 1989; Darby et al., 1995). According to Reebok Step Training Guidelines, beginners are easily and appropriately challenged at music speeds of 118–122 bpm. Safe cadences of 122–128 bpm are acceptable for participants at intermediate to advanced fitness levels seeking greater aerobic challenges. Table 2 shows the recommended platform heights and music speeds for different participant levels, from novice to advanced, based on research completed in 1996 (Scharff-Olson, et al.).

Table 2
Recommended platform heights and music speeds
for different participant levels

Participant Level	Platform Height*	Music Speed
Step 1: Novice Someone who has not taken part in a regular exercise class for some time.	4 inches	118–122 bpm
Step 2: Beginner A regular exerciser who has never done any step training.	up to 6 inches	124 bpm
Step 3: Intermediate A regular step trainer.	up to 8 inches	126 bpm
Step 4: Advanced A regular and skilled step trainer.	up to 10 inches	128 bpm

*Note: About 60 degrees of knee flexion during step exercise is preferable at all levels. Do not allow any participant to select a step height that requires the weightbearing knee to flex more than 90 degrees. (Reprinted with permission from Scharff-Olson & Miller, 1997.)

Mood Enhancement

Kennedy and Newton (1997) investigated the effect of step training exercise intensity on mood. Results after a series of step classes at high and low intensities revealed that tension, depression, fatigue, and anger decreased in both intensity groups, while vigor (a positive mood state) increased. Both high- and low-intensity step training in this study led to positive changes in mood.

Chapter Two

Choreographic Terminology

Step Reebok researchers developed universally accepted terms that all group fitness instructors should understand. An important consideration is step orientation, which is the relationship between the platform and the room. When teaching a class, traveling movements and directional changes should be cued using the orientations. The front of the room is where the instructor is standing. The sides refer to the two side walls, and the back refers to the back of the room. When participants face the instructor they are actually standing at the back of the platform, but are starting an approach called "from the front." Included below are definitions of various directional approaches to the platform itself, different acknowledged step movement types, and explanations for various step patterns.

Directional Approach

Directional approach describes the position of the body in relation to the platform, in preparation for a specific step movement pattern. There are six recognized approaches that can be of use in choreography design.

From the Front: Standing behind the platform, facing the front of the room or the instructor (Figure 2).

From the Side: Standing with one side of the body closer to the long edge of the platform. Moves from this approach are initiated sideways to the left or right from the side closest to the step (Figure 3).

Figure 2
From the Front
platform approach.

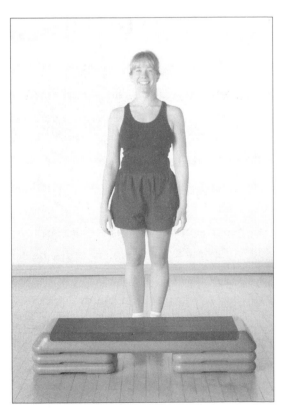

From the Corner: Similar to the From the Side approach, here the body is positioned at one corner of the long platform edge ready to initiate a move to the opposite diagonal corner (Figure 4).

From the Top: Standing on top of the platform, initiating movements down off the step (Figure 5).

From the End: Standing at one end of the platform facing the length of the step. This approach allows movements similar to those from the front or side, depending on body position when starting choreography from the end (Figure 6).

Astride: Standing on the floor straddling the platform. Movements are initiated upward onto the step (Figure 7).

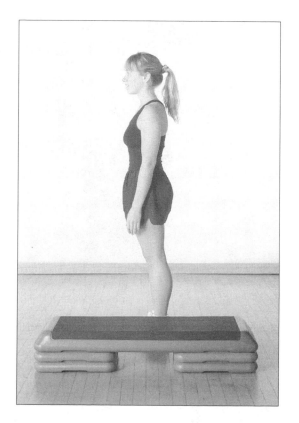

Figure 3
From the Side
platform
approach.

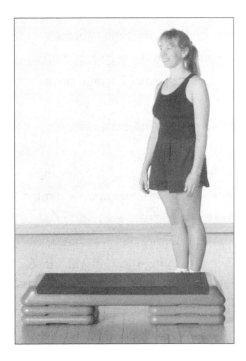

Figure 4
From the Corner
platform approach.

Figure 5
From the Top
platform approach.

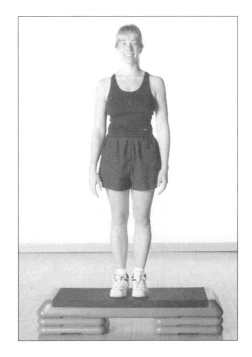

Figure 6
From the End
platform approach.

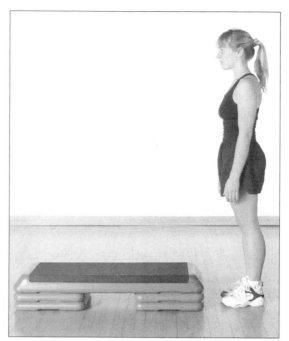

Figure 7
Astride
platform approach.

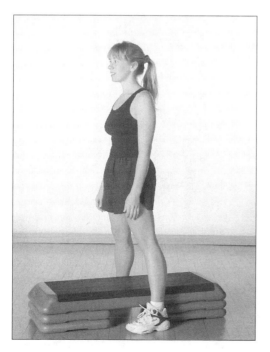

Step Types

There are a variety of step types available for use. As with directional approach, these are not names of movement patterns, but definitional terms that aid in the design of movement patterns.

Up Steps: Steps that start from the floor and step up onto the platform.

Down Steps: Steps that start from the top of the platform and step down to the floor.

Single Lead: Describes the same leg leading (initiating) each 4-count movement cycle.

Alternating Lead: Describes changing the lead foot every 4-count movement cycle.

Variations: Slightly different lever angle or movement that varies the previous basic step pattern.

Figure 8
Basic Step with a Right Lead Leg; Up (a.), Up (b.), Down (c.), Down.

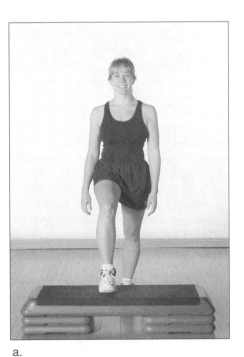

a.

Combinations: The linking together of different step patterns, combining any sequence of two or more directions and one or more step patterns.

Propulsions: Airborne steps, used to increase movement intensity, that may involve pivoting in the air.

Step Patterns

There are 21 different basic step patterns with specific terminology for use in movement cueing. The pattern names and movement descriptions are as follows:

Basic Step: Stepping up onto the platform then down in a 4-count movement of Up-Up-Down-Down. Can be Right Leg Lead or Left Leg Lead depending on which leg initiates the movement pattern, sometimes called "Basic Right" and "Basic Left," or "Right Basic" and "Left Basic" (Figure 8).

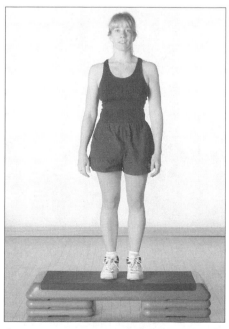
b.

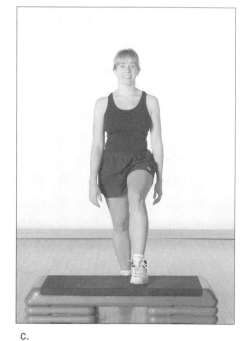
c.

V Step: Similar to the Basic Step, in this movement pattern the Up-Up portion of the 4-count movement involves placing the feet wide on either end of the platform. Then the Down-Down portion brings the feet together on the floor to complete a "V" formation. Also can be Right or Left Leg Leads, called "V Step Right/Left" or "Right/Left V Step" (Figure 9).

Tap Down: Although not used often as a movement cue, this term describes the action of one foot, which moves from the step to tap the floor, lightly touching the floor rather than

Figure 9
V Step end position after the first 2 counts of the 4-count move.

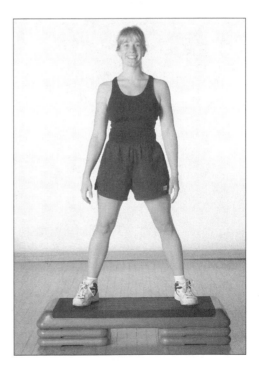

placing full body weight on the foot, and then lifts to initiate the next movement onto the step (Figure 10).

Tap Up: Similar to the Tap Down, in this move the action of the foot is to move from the floor and tap the step, lightly touching the platform without placing full body weight on the foot, then initiating the next move to the floor. A typical movement cycle would run Up-Tap-Down-Down (Figure 11).

Alternate Lead: This term describes changing lead legs with each movement cycle. Using the Tap Down move, an Alternate Lead is used with the Basic Step and V Step. Instructors some-

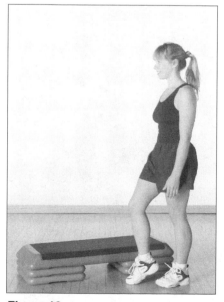

Figure 10
Tap Down
end position.

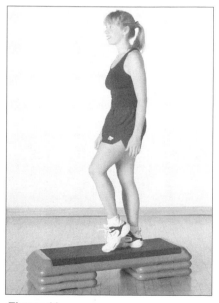

Figure 11
Tap Up
end position.

times say "Alternate Basic" or "Alternate V Step" to cue stepping Up-Up-Down-Tap 4-count movement cycles that change from right to left leg leads. Using the Tap Up move, an Alternate Lead allows the changing of lead legs to occur via the Tap Up onto the platform with the new lead leg initiating the step down to the floor.

Up Tap/Down Tap: This term describes the consecutive use of the Tap Up and Tap Down moves to create a single lead 4-count pattern. This is often used as a holding pattern for participants because it keeps them doing an easy movement that requires minimal stepping skill and does not alternate feet.

Figure 12

Over the Top movement; counts 1 (a.), 2 (b.), and 3 (c.).

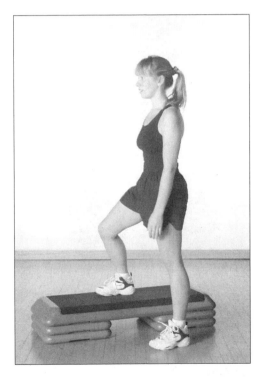

a.

Over the Top: This move involves traveling Over the Top of the platform using the Tap Down step. The approach begins from the Side, and the body remains facing that same side throughout the 4-count move. The first count moves the lead leg up onto the platform; next, the other leg lifts to the platform. Count 3 moves the lead leg onto the floor on the opposite side of the bench, and count 4 completes the move with a Tap Down of the leg on the step, which is ready to initiate the next move. In relation to traditional aerobics, this move is akin to two step-touches in one direction (Figure 12).

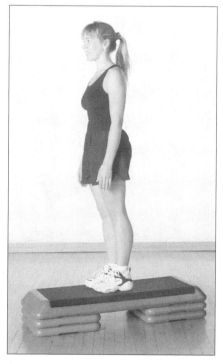

b.

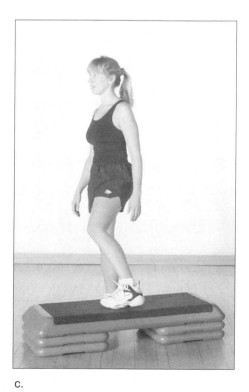

c.

A Step: This step skill can be performed from the Front or Side, as either a Single or Alternating Lead. From the Front, it begins near the edge of the platform and the first and second foot strikes are toward the center of the platform, to finish with a Tap Down on count 4 near the opposite edge of the

Figure 13
A Step, From the Front; counts 1 (a.), 2 (b.), and 3 (c.).

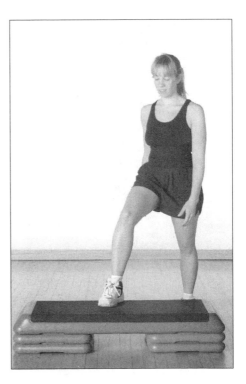

a.

platform. Essentially, this is a Basic Step that forms an A shape. From the Side, an A Step involves the first two foot strikes stepping slightly forward, and the last two slightly backward on the other side of the step. This move is essentially an Over The Top step that forms an A shape (Figure 13).

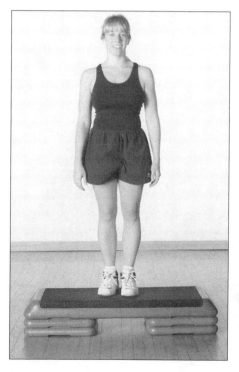

b.

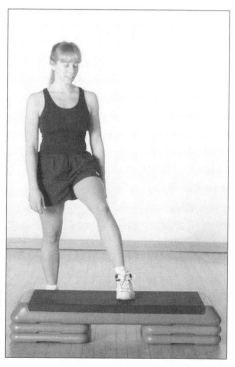

c.

Corner to Corner: This move involves traveling from one Corner of the platform to the opposite Corner in a diagonal motion, without stepping forward off the step (Figure 14).

Figure 14
Corner to Corner movement; counts 1 (a.), 2 (b.), and 3 (c.).

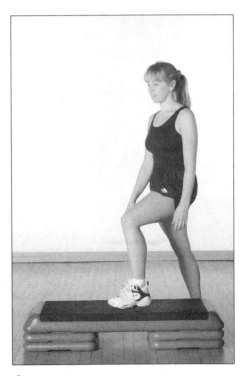

a.

Lift Steps (Single Lead): **This movement is a variation of the Tap Up where the foot that would tap the step instead performs a knee lift and then steps down to the floor for count 3 of a 4-

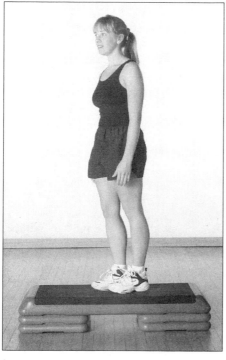

b.

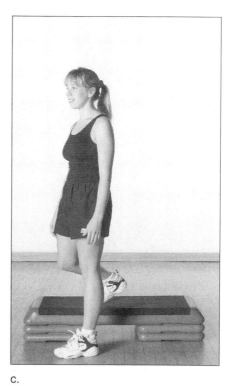

c.

count movement pattern. The lead leg completes count 4 in the pattern, performing either a Tap Down so the same leg can initiate the next move or a complete step so the other leg (which performed the knee lift) is ready to initiate the next movement. Variations include a kick, a leg abduction, and a hamstring curl (Figure 15).

Figure 15a
Lift Step movement; count 1.

Figure 15 b, c, & d
Variations for count 2 of a *Lift Step*; (b.) knee lift, (c.) leg abduction, and (d.) hamstring curl.

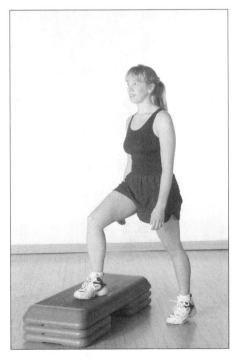

a.

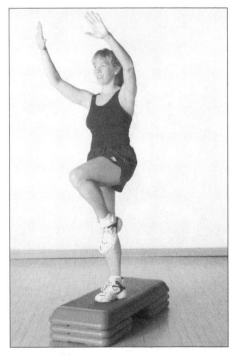

b.

Alternating Lift Steps: This term describes performing two or more consecutive knee lifts, kicks, leg curls, or leg abductions with an Alternate Lead. These moves can be performed from the Front, from the End, from Astride, or from the Top. For example, a Traveling Lift Step begins with a Front approach where the alternating lead move is used to angle the body toward each corner of

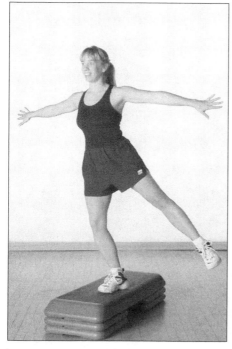

b.

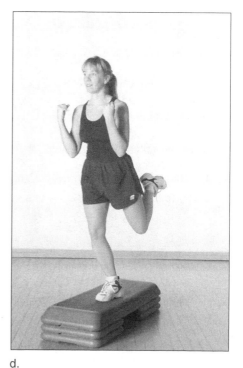

d.

the step in an Up-Knee lift-Down-Down pattern. The counts of each movement are changed with an approach beginning from the Top where the Alternating Lift Step would begin with the step down from the platform in a Down-Down-Up-Knee lift pattern.

Repeater: This is a higher intensity 8-count movement cycle where one leg repeats a specified move three consecutive times, while body weight remains centered over the stabilizing lead leg, which is planted on the step throughout the repeated movement. The repeated move can be a knee lift (Knee Repeater), kick (Kick Repeater), leg curl (Hamstring Repeater), or leg abduction

Figure 16
A *Repeater* involves stepping onto the platform (a.) and repeating a *Lift Step* (b.) three times in a row while the Lead Leg stays weightbearing and the Lifting Leg Taps the floor between Lift Steps (c.).

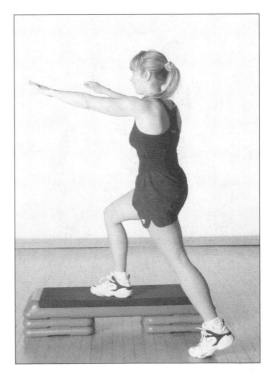

a.

(Abduction Repeater). Knee Repeater example (beginning on the right leg): count 1 of the 8-count cycle, right leg steps up onto the platform; count 2, left leg performs the first knee lift; count 3, left leg taps down on the floor lightly; count 4, repeat the knee lift; count 5, tap the floor again; count 6, complete the third knee lift of the Repeater; count 7, left leg to the floor; count 8, right leg Taps Down or completely steps down to allow the other leg to initiate the next move (Figure 16). Note that Repeaters can be choreographed in different numbers (i.e., 2-knee Repeater, or 5-

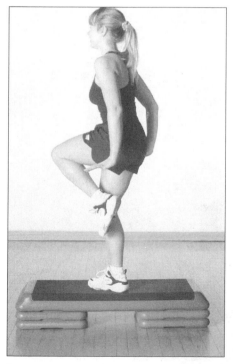

b.

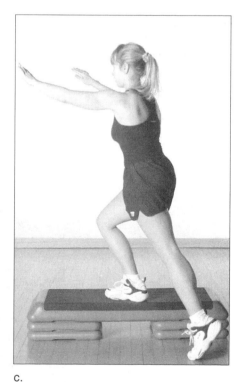

c.

curl Repeater), but more than five should never be consecutively performed, and the standard definition involves three repetitions of a movement.

Turn Step: Also called a Travel Step and a Traveling Tap Down, this 4-count movement can be described as a Basic Step that involves externally rotating the hips to turn the body toward the center of the room on the Tap Down. The platform is approached from the Side (one side of the body closer to the step, facing one of the side walls or corner of the room), with the first

Figure 17a
A *Turn Step* begins count 1 from the Side, stepping up onto the platform with the Lead Leg angled toward the Front.

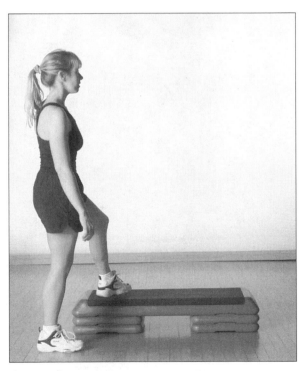

a.

step up onto the platform turning the body from facing the Side/Corner to facing Front with a slightly angled leg. The next step up onto the platform has the other leg angling so the body turns toward the other Side or Corner. The final Tap Down places the opposite side of the body closest to the platform ready to initiate the next move with the opposite lead leg. Note that although the body turns, it remains on the same side of the platform (Figure 17). Additionally, Turn Steps are completed with

Figure 17 b & c
The *Turn Step* continues with a weight shift atop the platform facing Front (b.), then steps down so the other side of the body is closest to the platform (c.).

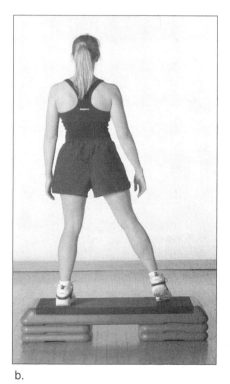

b.

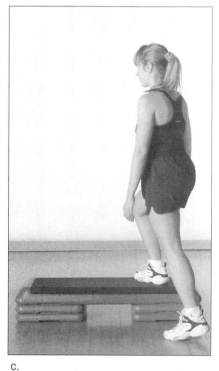

c.

either a Right Lead or Left Lead, and are sometimes cued as "Right Turn" or "Left Turn."

Straddle Down: This move begins from the Top of the platform, facing either End. The 4-count move is completed by first stepping down to straddle the bench (counts 1 and 2), then returning up to the platform for counts 3 and 4 with the lead leg first, for a Down-Down-Up-Up pattern. On count 4 the non-lead leg returning to the step can perform a Tap Up, so that leg is ready to initiate the next move. If a Tap Up is completed and another Straddle Down

Figure 18a
The starting position for the *Straddle Down* movement.

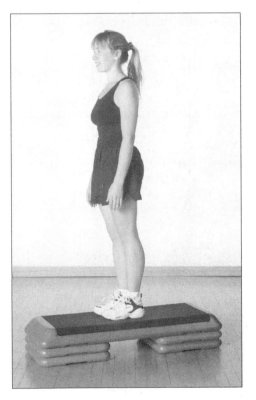

a.

with the other lead leg is done, this is an Alternate Straddle Down. Sometimes this move is called "Straddle Right" or "Straddle Left," describing which leg leads each Straddle Down move (Figure 18).

Straddle Up: This move is exactly opposed to the Straddle Down. It begins from Astride the platform, steps Up-Up onto the bench, then returns Down-Down Astride the bench. The 4-count pattern can end here also with a complete step or a Tap Down,

Figure 18b & c
Counts 1 (b.) and 2 (c.) of the
Straddle Down movement.

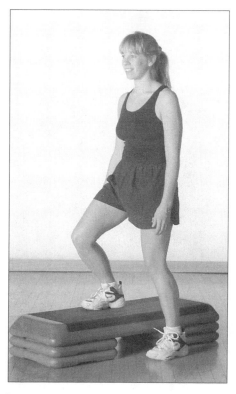

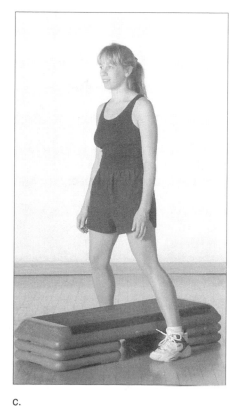

b.

c.

creating an Alternate Straddle Up that mimics the Alternating Basic Step.

Across the Top (Lateral): This high-intensity move mimics the Over the Top move with a different starting position. The 4-count Across the Top pattern begins from the End of the platform, facing the Front of the room. The step moves the body

Figure 19

Across the Top begins with a lateral Step Up to the platform from the Side on either End (a.), continues laterally with a propulsive weight shift (b.), and ends with a Step Down to the other End (c.).

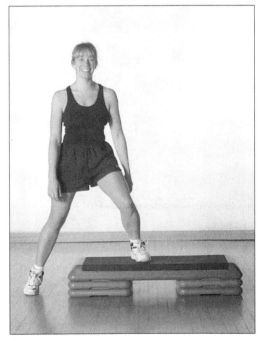

a.

across the length of the platform with a slight propulsion (depending on leg length and step height) to finish in the same position on the opposite End of the platform. As it is a lateral move, this is sometimes called Lateral Across. Critical for this movement skill is that participants take a big enough first step up so they can keep their hips level as they lift onto and travel across the platform (Figure 19).

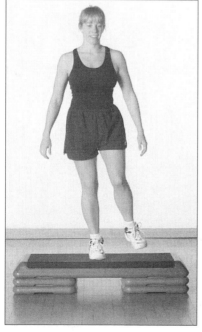

b.

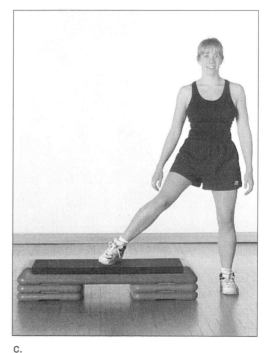

c.

L Step: This 8-count movement is easily described with Tap Ups and Tap Downs, but is usually used with Lift Steps. Using the Right Leg Lead as the example, on count 1 the right leg steps up on the platform close to one End. On count 2 the left leg Taps Up on the step, on count 3 the left leg Taps Down to the side of the platform, and on count 4 the right leg Taps Down next to the left, placing the body in a "from the end" approach facing the Front of the room. The next four counts that complete the L Step simply reverse what has just been completed. On count 5 the right leg

Figure 20
The *L Step* begins from the Front toward one End of the platform (a.). Counts 2 (b.), 3 (c.), and 4 (d.) of the *L Step* using knee lifts; the remaining 4 counts of the *L Step* simply reverse the first 4 to return to the start position.

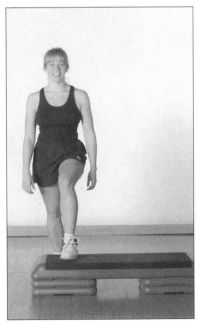

a.

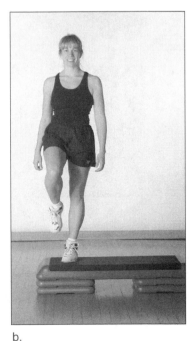

b.

(closest to the platform) Taps Up, on count 6 the left leg Taps Up, and on count 7 the left leg Taps Down backward to the floor. On count 8 the right leg Taps or steps down to fully return the body to the beginning position with a Front approach. This easily leads into an L Step on the other End of the platform. When two alternating L steps are completed the 16-count move is sometimes called a W Step. To add intensity, knee lifts may be added in place of each Tap (Figure 20).

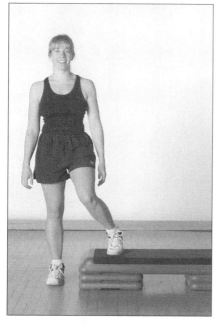

c.

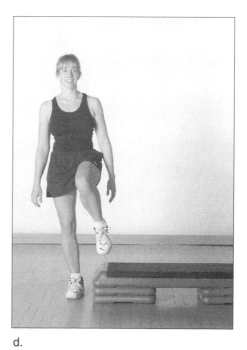

d.

T Step: This 8-count move begins from either End of the platform, facing that End. Described with a right leg lead, on count 1 the right leg steps up. On count 2 the left leg steps up, on count 3 the right leg straddles the platform, and on count 4 the left leg straddles the other side of the platform to create the Astride approach. On count 5 the right leg steps up to the

Figure 21
The *T Step* begins facing one End of the platform (a.). Counts 2 (b.), 3 (c.), and 4 (d.) place the participant Astride the platform. Counts 5 (e.), 6 (f.), and 7 (g.) finish the *T Step* by reversing the first 4 counts to return to the platform End.

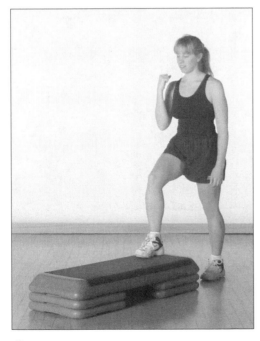

a.

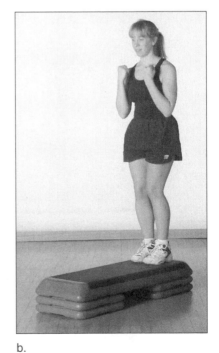

b.

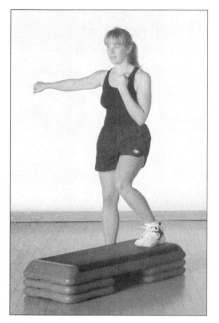

c.

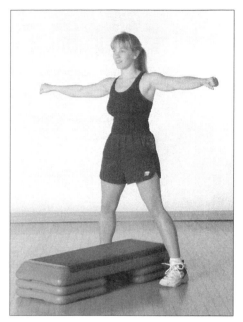

d.

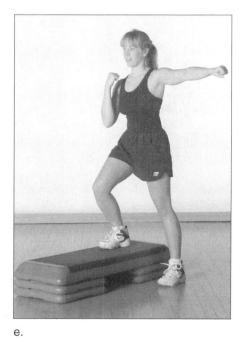

e.

platform again. On count 6 the left leg steps up, on count 7 the right leg steps down backward, and on count 8 the left leg steps down backward to return the body to the start position from the End of the step. Easy cueing for the T Step might sound something like "Up-Up-Straddle-Straddle-Up-Up-Off the Back" (Figure 21).

Figure 21
(continued)

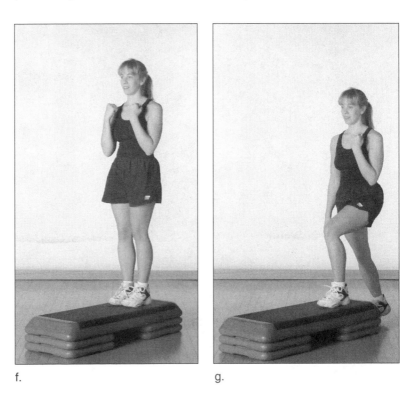

f.   g.

U Turn: This direction-changing move can be thought of as a "small turn step," and involves completing a Turn Step using half of the platform with a Tap Down on count 4 to change lead legs. It is especially effective around a Corner, when changing from an End to Side or a Side to End approach (Figure 22).

Figure 22
The *U Turn* looks like a Turn Step on a small portion of the platform.

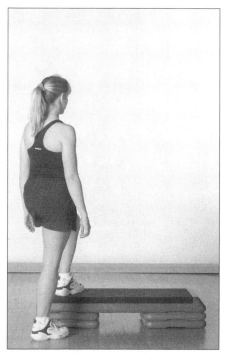

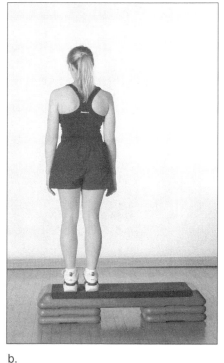

a.

b.

Lunges: These are high-intensity movements that take place from the Top of the step facing either the Front (lunges are performed directly backwards) or Side (lunges are performed laterally off the platform). A lunge is really a 2-count move that requires one leg to remain stable on the platform while the other lunges to lightly Tap Down on the floor and then return to the platform. Most lunges are performed as "singles," which

Figure 22
(continued)

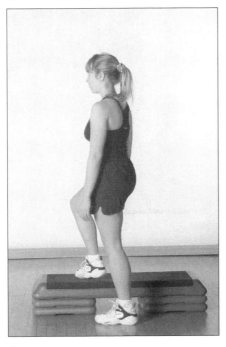

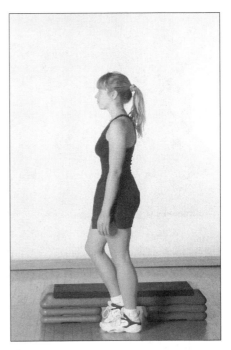

c.

d.

alternate the lunging legs. Variations for increased challenge include two and four lunges on one leg. Throughout the lunge, body weight must remain on the stabilizing leg, rather than transferring to the lunging leg. Lunges are advanced moves that need to be performed with great control (Figure 23). Parallel Squat Lunges are another way to increase intensity. Essentially a half-tempo Lunge, Parallel Squats take place from atop the step facing

Figure 23a
Lunge from the Top facing the End of the platform.

Figure 23b
Lunge from the Top facing Front.

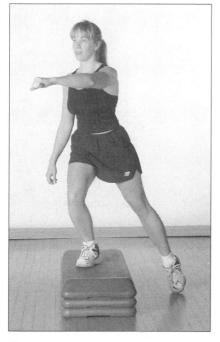

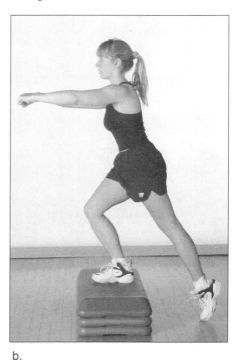

a.

b.

either End. They involve placing the entire foot laterally on the floor to squat, with the body weight evenly distributed (Figure 24).

Hop Turns: Also called Pop Turns, these propulsive movements require airborne shifting of body weight. The 4-count move involves the lead leg stepping up to the platform and leaping into the air to turn the body (count 1), landing on the step in a new position (count 2), the other leg held lifted during the airborne move steps down to the floor (count 3), and lastly the lead leg steps to the floor.

Figure 24
A *Squat* from atop the step is a high-intensity, half-time Lunge variation.

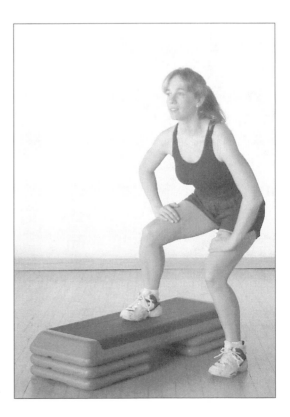

Hop Turns can take place at the corner of the platform, involving a 90 degree rotation of the body while in mid-air (a ¼ Hop Turn), or across the platform from front to back involving a 180 degree rotation of the body while in mid-air (a ½ Hop Turn). Note that the ¼ Hop Turn is less difficult because it involves less movement and rotation. Hop Turns must never be performed unless the body weight is entirely lifted into the air (Figure 25).

Figure 25
Hop Turns involve the airborne shifting of body weight.

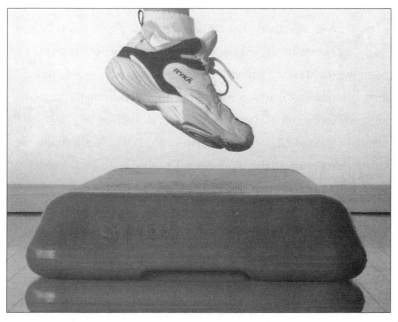

Chapter Three

Kinesiology

Vertical Impact Forces

Since its inception, step training has been praised as a high-fitness, relatively low-impact activity. Numerous studies have evaluated the effectiveness of different step-training movements, demonstrating that non-propulsive step patterns produce sufficient cardiorespiratory demands for improving aerobic fitness (Calarco et al., 1991; Francis et al., 1991; Scharff-Olson et al., 1991; Stanforth et al., 1993). Non-propulsive movements such as the Basic Step Up-Up-Down-Down on a moderately high bench of 6 to 8 inches yield impact forces of 1.4 to 1.5 times body weight (averaging all four foot strikes in the Basic step), similar to the impact of brisk walking (Francis, 1992). Additionally, early step research that examined basic stepping at 120 bpm on a 10-inch platform determined that the first leg to step down from the platform on any 4-count step cycle has the greatest vertical impact force, averaging 1.75 times body weight (Francis et al., 1990).

Much like faster speeds when jogging, propulsive techniques substantially increase the intensity of step training, and create impact forces similar to those seen with jogging or high-impact aerobic dance exercise, averaging 2.5 times body weight (Michaud et al., 1993; Olson & Williford, 1998). These movements should be offered on a limited basis in any class, and reserved exclusively for intermediate to advanced exercisers. Propulsive, or power, moves should never be performed down onto the floor, but rather only up onto the platform, which is resilient and absorbs impact.

Fatigue and Stability

Repeaters and Lunges are movements used to increase the intensity of step training. The standard definition of a Repeater involves three repetitions of a Lift Step, and more than five should never be consecutively performed. Similarly, five consecutive lunges on one leg should never be performed. The reasoning behind this guideline is that both of these high-intensity movements involve repetitive loading to the stabilizing or base leg on the platform. As the number of repetitions increases, the loaded leg becomes more fatigued and less stable, compromising form and creating potential for injury. For these same reasons, single lead step movements (Basic Step, V Step, Tap Up/Down, Straddle Up/Down, and Lift Steps) should be performed consecutively for no more than one minute on the same leg.

Knee Compression Forces

Anytime the knee flexes, the patella contacts the femur and is guided through the movement by a patello-femoral groove, formed by rounded projections on the femur. The patella and femur are lined by articular cartilage that prevents these bones from rubbing against each other. A loaded (weightbearing) and flexed knee joint places compression forces on the back of the kneecap that increase as flexion progresses and are further accelerated if kneecap tracking is misaligned. Studies have revealed that kneecap compression forces are only slightly more than body weight when the knee is flexed to 60 degrees from the fully extended position, increasing swiftly as deeper flexion occurs, especially beyond 90 degrees (Reilly & Martens, 1972). Step training involves placing weight on a flexed knee, when the lead leg is placed on the platform and body weight shifts so the other leg can be lifted off the floor. Large compressive forces may over time cause the protective cartilage between the patella and femur to soften, become rough or frayed, or crack and blister. This erosion of cartilage then allows the patella to directly rub against the femur, possibly causing severe pain. To avoid this, platform heights should be chosen to restrict loading of the knee joint to 90 degrees at most, while 60 degrees or less is recommended for more biomechanical safety and comfort.

Spinal and Foot Alignment

During step training posture should be aligned so that movements take place with a full-body lean from the ankles (Figure 26). This is a naturally occurring position when stepping up and down, due to the tendency to main-

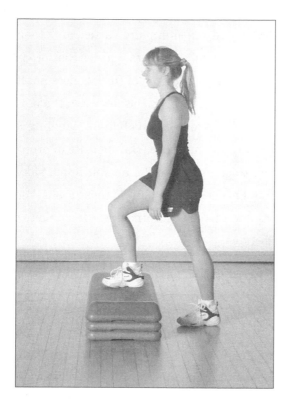

Figure 26
A full-body
lean; the
correct step
posture.

tain center of gravity over the lead leg for balance. Instruct participants not to lean from the waist (forward, backward, or sideways) during step exercise. Leaning from the waist can stress the low back, as uneven compression of the intervertebral disks is created by the weight of the head, trunk, and arms. The spine can be further stressed when spinal muscles have to forcibly contract to keep the body from falling forward.

Participants that pronate or supinate significantly enough to experience pain should be advised to seek expert assistance. Pronation, motion where the foot flattens and the tibia turns toward the midline of the body, naturally occurs to provide shock absorption in the ideal foot structure. However, overstretched foot muscles and ligaments can create a flattened arch during weightbearing exercise, causing shin pain. Participants that pronate excessively are more vulnerable to injuries that produce knee pain. Supination, where the arch of the foot does not flatten sufficiently to support body weight, occurs when the muscles and ligaments of the foot are excessively tight, yielding high arches. Participants that supinate (the opposite of pronation) are less able to cushion impact and transmit impact forces to the shins, hips, and back, causing pain in those areas. Fortunately, proper shoes and in-shoe orthotics are often able to correct foot imperfections.

Muscle Involvement

In step exercise, the main muscles involved in movement, the primary movers, are those in the lower body. The abdominals and erector spinae are stabilizers of the torso during step training, and maintaining appropriate tension in these muscle groups is critical for holding proper form throughout an exercise session. It is the lower-body musculature however, that generates and controls movement during step exercises. Table 3 lists the major lower-body muscles used in step training, along with their primary actions. Each of these muscles contracts at different times and in different amounts to perform the various movements patterns used in step training.

Table 3
Lower-body muscles used in step training and their primary actions

MUSCLE	JOINT	ACTION
Iliacus	Hip	hip flexion and lateral rotation
Psoas major and psoas minor	Hip	hip flexion and lateral rotation
Rectus femoris	Hip	hip flexion
Rectus femoris	Knee	knee extension
Gluteus maximus	Hip	hip extension, abduction, adduction, and lateral rotation
Gluteus medius and gluteus minimus	Hip	hip abduction
Biceps femoris	Hip	hip extension and lateral rotation
Biceps femoris	Knee	knee flexion and lateral rotation
Semitendinosus	Hip	hip extension
Semitendinosus	Knee	knee flexion and medial rotation
Semimembranosus	Hip	hip extension
Semimembranosus	Knee	knee flexion and medial rotation
Adductor magnus	Hip	hip adduction and lateral rotation
Adductor brevis and longus	Hip	adduction, flexion, and medial rotation
Vastus medialis, intermedius, and lateralis	Knee	knee extension
Anterior tibialis	Ankle	ankle dorsiflexion; foot inversion
Peroneus longus	Ankle	ankle plantarflexion; foot eversion
Peroneus brevis	Ankle	ankle plantarflexion; foot eversion
Gastrocnemius	Ankle	ankle plantarflexion
Soleus	Ankle	ankle plantarflexion

Chapter Four

Teaching a Step Class

G roup fitness instructors are obligated to teach participants proper step techniques while providing a safe stepping environment and class format. Alignment is critically important in step training. Participants must be advised to keep the back straight, chest and head up, and the buttocks and abdomen contracted. Shoulders should remain aligned over the hips to prevent a forward lean from the waist, and a whole-body lean from the ankles should be encouraged. Additionally, the knees must be kept aligned over the feet when pulling the body weight up onto the platform. Knees should be kept "soft," with a slight bend as opposed to locking the knee joint, when the legs are straightened. Steps up onto the platform should be light, with the entire foot being placed solidly on the platform and the heel bearing the weight. Steps down should be close to the platform, landing on the toe/ball of the foot, then bringing the heel completely down to the floor (propulsion and lunge steps excluded).

Participants should regularly glance at their platform, especially if they are inexperienced, deconditioned, or learning a new movement pattern.

Verbal Introduction

The beginning of every step class should include a welcome by the instructor and a brief description of the class, along with the identification of participants new to step training or new to your class. Further, risk assessment of all participants should be done to determine appropriateness of the step activity for each, along with a review of proper stepping techniques. Offer a review of intensity-monitoring techniques, as well as recommended modifications in step training.

Equipment

For a traditional step training class, the main component needed is a step product or wood bench (Figure 27). Recommended dimensions are 6 to 8 inches high by 12 inches wide by 24 to 36 inches long. Height adjustments are ideal, so participants can begin at an appropriate level and progress as fitness gains are made. Most platforms are 4 inches high at their lowest, with height adjustments in 2-inch increments. In addition to adjustable heights, a good platform will have a nonslip surface, rounded and smooth edges and corners, and be of full size. Mini-models are available, but are not recommended because they limit the size of movement patterns available and are potentially hazardous because they are easier to fall off. Further, a good platform will not sag or wobble when stood upon.

Figure 27a
4-inch platform.

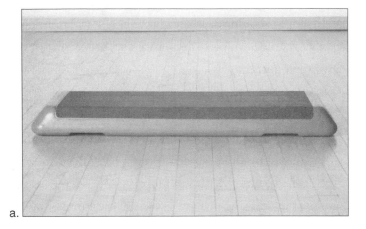

a.

Figure 27b
6-inch platform.

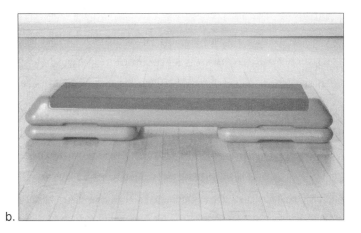

b.

Figure 27c
8-inch platform.

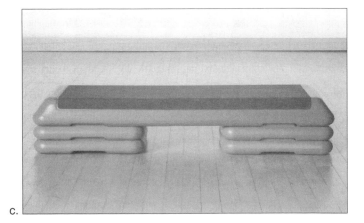

c.

Cueing

The most crucial factor in leading an enjoyable group exercise class is effective, timely cueing. If cues are not delivered correctly participants will not have a good experience in class. Cueing is even more critical in step classes because a poorly timed or improperly worded cue may cause participants to miss a step on the platform and injure themselves.

Cues are the signals that mark the beginning of a thought or action and serve as a warning system that allows participants to follow a movement pattern easily. Your ability to effectively cue a movement change to a class determines the success of the participants, and when done properly ensures them a smooth and continuous aerobic workout. Three types of cues are used in a group exercise class:

- *Movement cues* simply describe a movement to be done and when that move begins. Example: "L Step Right in 4, 3, 2..."
- *Safety and alignment cues* are very important in step training, where form is so important for injury prevention. These cues are reminders or corrections to movements already taking place or about to begin. Example: "Lean from the ankles rather than bending at the waist."
- *Motivational cues* are provided to add energy to a class setting, creating an environment where participants feel good about performing the exercise. Example: "Excellent form everyone, you're doing great!"

For instructors new to teaching or new to a particular exercise modality, movement cues are most important. Once movement cues have become second nature, safety and motivational cueing should be utilized regularly. An easy way to deliver movement cues is to consider three things: body part, action, and direction. A cue should tell participants what body part will be changing (arms/leg/muscle group), what action that body part will be doing (curling, lifting), and in which direction the action will occur (front/back, to the right/left). Other information that clarifies the movement can be added, but the above items are critical to provide participants with information to execute the movement pattern change appropriately.

> Effective cues are given in the 4 counts prior to movement execution, preceding the change. For example, if a movement change is planned from two basic right leads to alternating knee lifts the cue would be given during the 4 counts of the second basic step. It is helpful also to finish the cue with one beat to spare, ending the cue before the movement begins so participants have time to process the information of the cue and begin execution.

Some of the step-training moves have more than one accepted term ("Turn Step" or "Travel Step"). Make certain that once a cue is chosen for a move, that term is used every time. Changing words and phrases only adds confusion and detracts from the exercise experience. Further, many instructors that teach step training have developed names that represent a specific sequence of movements ("Indecision" or "Popcorn," etc.). Make certain when substituting for another instructor's class that base movements are cued, rather than using the specific names used with regular participants.

Voice inflection can motivate and add energy to the class setting. Cues should begin somewhat softer and lower, and build up to louder and higher to drive participants toward action, creating a sense of urgency.

Use of visual cues minimizes the need for verbal cues, aiding in voice protection while assisting with communication to participants in large classes or in rooms with poor acoustics or no microphone. Visual cues should be as consistent as verbal cues, timed to end one beat before the movement, be sharp and clean, and be visible, overhead whenever possible. Examples of visual cues in step training include a circular motion with one arm overhead to indicate a turn step, or patting the top of the head to indicate that a combination or movement pattern will be repeated from the top.

Intensity Monitoring

Encourage participants to pace themselves throughout a step class, monitoring fatigue to avoid injury. The Rating of Perceived Exertion method for assessing work level can be explained and used while participants are stepping. When a heart rate measurement is taken, encourage students to consult a posted heart rate chart to evaluate exercise intensity.

Injury Prevention

Group fitness instructors should, at all times, have injury prevention uppermost in their minds. Proper execution of step movements and proper form during activity provide participants with the opportunity for years of participation and enjoyment.

Biomechanics

The best way to avoid injury from step training is to practice all of the guidelines outlined in this book. One of the most important factors in injury prevention is step height.

Guide participants to choose a step height that is appropriately challenging without compromising form. Researchers have established that joint reaction forces and contact pressures at the patello-femoral joint increase considerably as loaded knee flexion angles increase. Platform heights that require knee flexion greater than 90 degrees significantly compress the knee joint, possibly leading to premature degeneration of patella articular cartilage and the overuse injury called patella pain syndrome (Reilly & Martens, 1972). Requa et al. (1993) reported 10 knee injuries or complaints of knee pain for each 1,000 hours of participation in step training, demonstrating that the knee is a common injury site and preventative measures are called for to minimize stress to this joint.

Hoose et al. (1998) examined the clinical relevance of knee flexion during step training and determined that step height, total body weight, and femur length all affect knee joint flexion angle. Their recommendation upon kinematic analysis of the knee joint during stepping, is to select a step height based on limb length versus fitness level. They further concluded that minimizing loaded knee flexion angles decreases the risk of patellar cartilage degeneration. At 90 degrees of flexion the knee is loaded with slightly more than three times body weight, and at 60 degrees the load is approximately equal to body weight. Researchers determined that the least amount of knee compression occurred at 30 degrees of loaded knee flexion (Figure 28).

Although the use of a 4- to 6-inch platform (causing 30 degrees or less of knee flexion for the majority of adults) as the standard step height for most participants seeking fitness gains is unlikely, there is another way to minimize stress on the knee joint caused by step training. Encourage participants to supplement

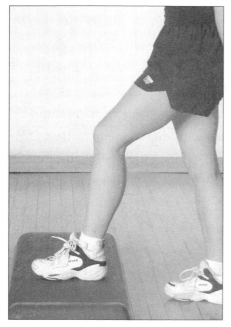

a.

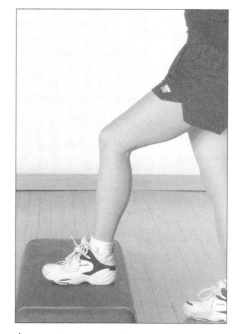

b.

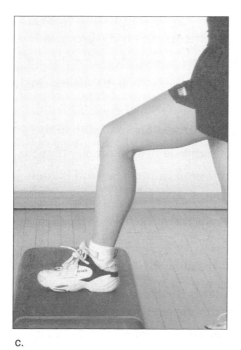

c.

Figure 28
Increasing degrees of
knee flexion as step height
increases from 4 inches
(a.) to 6 inches (b.) and
8 inches (c.).

their step training exercise program with an activity that does not involve stepping up and down (e.g., a stair climber or step mill), but rather an activity utilizing different muscle groups and/or a different movement pattern, such as walking, swimming, or cycling. In this manner regular steppers can best prevent overuse injuries associated with step training, such as chondromalacia. Individuals with chronic knee problems are advised to avoid step training as it is most likely not a suitable activity for them.

Other overuse injuries commonly seen in step training relate to improper stepping form. Stepping too far back from the platform (more than one shoe length away) creates a slight forward lean of the body that stresses the foot, Achilles', and calf, possibly causing Achilles' tendonitis (Figure 29). This condition may also be seen with repetitive stepping up to the platform with heels hanging over the edge (not placing the entire foot on the platform). Such a forward body lean also interferes with the ability to maintain neutral posture during step. Bouncing on the toes when stepping — not allowing the entire foot to be placed on the floor when stepping down off the platform — concentrates the impact forces of step in the forefoot area (Figure 30). This can lead to arch problems such as plantar fasciitis, a painful overuse injury that can become a chronic condition.

Stepping heavily is also a common problem in step training. Often caused by music speed that is too fast or poor stepping technique, heavy stepping can result in an increase in the impact forces of step training with the body less able to compensate and absorb impact stress. Greater impact stress due to vertical forces during step training equates to greater risk of injury.

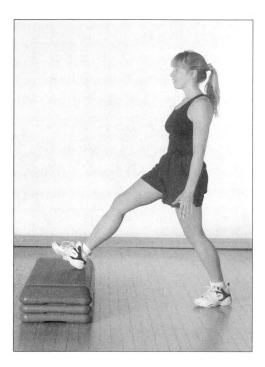

Figure 29
Improper stepping
technique; stepping
too far back from
the platform.

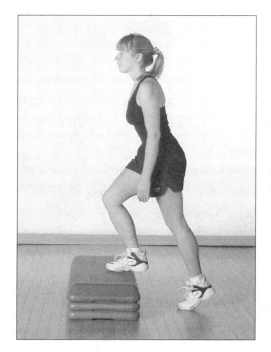

Figure 30
Improper stepping
technique; stepping
with heels hanging
off the platform
edge (heels do not
contact the
platform) and
bouncing on the
toes (heels do not
contact the floor).

Vertical impact forces have been examined by investigators and are related directly to step height and step speed, ranging from 1.4 to 1.7 times body weight for the basic step pattern on 6- and 10-inch platforms at 120 bpm (Johnson et al., 1993). Higher impact power moves like lunges, repeaters, or propulsion steps generate forces 1.9 to 2.9 times body weight on 6- to 12-inch platforms at 120–132 bpm (Scharff-Olson et al., 1996). Interestingly, the Scharff-Olson study found experienced steppers able to control movements and dissipate impact forces with greater ability than novices, indicating that step experience appears to teach a force-absorbing response that minimizes risk of injury. To ensure the development of such skill, however, the authors concluded participants need to begin on a lower platform height at slower step speeds, increasing both only after an adjustment period.

A suitable shoe for step training is also important for injury prevention. Step exercise requires a shoe with an adequate heel lift that reduces the calf and Achilles' stresses. Additionally, step shoes need good forefoot flexibility to accommodate the toe-ball-heel and toe-strike-only landings associated with step movement patterns. Running shoes are inappropriate due to the lack of freedom of movement allowed on some platform surfaces. Shoes specifically designed for step training, cross-trainers, and some aerobics shoes offer a wider, more stable heel and the needed forefoot cushion. One other important consideration for shoes that will be used in step training is an Achilles' "notch." This downward curve in the back edge of a shoe allows for complete dorsi- and plantarflexion through the ankles' full range of motion, without placing friction or pressure on the Achilles' tendon in mid- or high-top shoes.

A study of common injuries among step training instructors revealed that most injuries are low-grade and are related to muscle soreness. Compared to running and traditional aerobic dance, step training carries a lower risk of serious injury (Scharff-Olson et al., 1996). Overall, it appears that step exercise does not pose a greater risk of injury than traditional dance exercise formats, but the injury sites seen with step training are different.

Environment

The appropriate environment for step training is similar to that of any group exercise class, including a supportive floor, space for movement, and proper ventilation. Additionally, appropriate step equipment is necessary (see Equipment, page 51). Mirrors in a classroom are extremely helpful in step training, but not necessary.

"Mirroring" participants, or facing the class when teaching, creates a comfortable, welcoming environment that allows you to make eye contact with each participant. With step training, however, this is difficult for many movement patterns that do not directly face the front of the room. Once a movement pattern crosses over the top of the platform or involves straddling, for example, participants become confused as to the appropriate position of their feet and body. It is advisable to face the same direction as the class during more complex movement patterns and clearly point out to participants when mirroring is taking place to minimize risk of participant injury should they try to suddenly alter their foot pattern to match your "mirrored" position.

Another facet to class environment that affects injury prevention during step training involves the atmosphere created by the instructor. Seek to create a non-judgmental environment that is fun and non-competitive. In this way, participants will feel comfortable modifying step movement patterns and even selecting platform heights that meet their individual needs. High-pressure, competitive atmospheres where participants feel too intimidated to make appropriate decisions for their fitness needs place them in danger of injury. For this reason, provide and encourage the use of movement options during step, and also make sure participants do not feel obligated to step at any specific platform height.

Personal Limitations

Instruct participants to follow their individual health and fitness limitations related to step training. People with chronic knee and/or lower back problems are most likely suited for a different activity. Individuals who are older, deconditioned, or of less than average height should remain at a step height of 6 inches or below. Additionally, steppers who are older, deconditioned, highly overweight, or unskilled are advised to participate in step classes taught at slower speeds, and avoid propulsion movements, which increase impact and require advanced movement skills. Those with any health limitations, from orthopedic to cardiac conditions, after obtaining a physician's release to exercise, should also step at slower speeds on low platform heights and avoid high-intensity, high-impact movements such as propulsions. Fitness level can be another limiting factor during step, and participants should monitor fatigue carefully as it compromises form and can lead to injury.

Modifications

After attending a number of step classes, exercisers will experience the fitness adaptations that come with regular participation in any aerobic modality, and therefore become more fit at stepping. Basic movements and lower step heights that once elicited higher-intensity physiological responses become easier to perform and less fatiguing. Many instructors and participants respond to this by increasing the intensity of stepping by increasing platform height, using faster music, performing more complex choreography, or holding hand weights or wearing ankle/wrist weights.

You are responsible for ensuring that participants receive a workout that is both safe and effective. Be aware of the biomechanical risks associated with each of the above modifications and guide participants to make appropriate decisions regarding use of those modifications.

Hand Weights

The use of hand-held weights (or ankle and wrist weights) during step training is a controversial issue (Figure 31). When step training first began, Kravitz and Deivert (1992) studied the use of hand weights. The information on increasing intensity recommended the use of "light hand weights of one or two pounds, if you can keep your alignment correct and your moves controlled." While still true that alignment must be correct and movements controlled when using hand weights, a variety of research has been conducted to determine the effects of hand weight use while stepping.

Preliminary studies on the effectiveness of hand-held weights during step yielded interesting results. Scharff-Olson et al. (1991)

Figure 31
Discourage the use of hand weights while stepping.

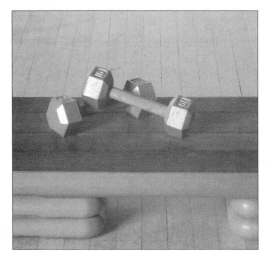

studied the cardiovascular and metabolic effects of step training in females, including the physiological response to using 1- and 2-pound hand weights while stepping on an 8-inch platform. Hand weights of 2 pounds resulted in the additional energy expenditure of only 1 kcal/min. Further, subjects stepping with 2-pound weights in the study complained of acute muscle pain and soreness during the exercise routine. The authors concluded that participants should seek to increase the energy expenditure of step training through other means.

In 1993, Kravitz et al. examined the physiological effects of stepping with and without hand-held weights (0.5 to 1.5 pounds) over an eight-week training period. Arm movements mirrored leg movements for both groups, including controlled motions for the entire 30-minute step exercise routine. Similar improvements were reported for both the hand-weight and non-hand-weight groups for oxygen uptake, body composition, and muscularity. Subjects who trained with hand weights also reported notable amounts of upper-body muscular fatigue in the limbs and torso after 30 minutes of step training.

Kravitz et al. (1997) revisited the issue, looking at the training effects of hand weights on step exercise over a 12-week training period. Here again both training groups (with and without 2- to 3-pound hand weights) experienced similar improvements in body composition, muscular strength, and maximal oxygen uptake. No upper-body injuries were reported for either group in this study, and the authors concluded that step training with hand weights, similar to without hand weights, positively effects the cardiorespiratory system without additional risk of injury. Of note however, is that the hand weight group in this study progressed over their 12-week training period from no weights, to 2-pound, 2.5-pound, and finally 3-pound weights. Exercises were performed with weights for 12 to 15 minutes (versus the 30 minutes of the earlier study), and involved specific controlled motions very unlike the typical energetic pumping of the arms seen in group exercise. The controlled arm movements required with the use of hand weights are, the authors propose, not vigorous enough to increase energy expenditure or relative intensity of step aerobic training beyond that of exercise without hand weights.

Participants seeking to use weights during step training often want to increase intensity by performing the same arm movements they would without hand weights. This is extremely dangerous and greatly increases injury risk to the shoulder girdle based on research conducted on the use of hand weights during aerobic dance (Williford et al., 1989). Heavier weights result in significant fatigue and soreness when moved rapidly through full ranges of motion, creating great biomechanical risk of injury. Overall, the increase in energy expenditure seen with the proper use of hand weights during step training is minimal. Light weights do not provide the stimulus needed to see muscle definition or muscle hypertrophy; further, movements must be controlled and their use limited to avoid injury. Hand weights should be reserved for muscle-strengthening segments of the step class where movements are designed to be performed in a slow and controlled manner. The use of ankle or wrist weights should be discouraged, as the benefits are minimal at most and risk of injury is greatly increased when weights are used improperly.

Torso Weights

The results of adding torso weights while step training have also been examined (Stanforth & Stanforth, 1996). External scuba weights in 3-pound, 6-pound, and 9-pound increments added to the waist of step exercisers yielded increases in aerobic (oxygen uptake and heart rate) requirements. Results indicated that the aerobic requirements of step training are affected by adding external weight to the torso as if it were additional body weight. Increasing external weight by 20 pounds is equivalent to a 2-inch increase in platform height, increasing stepping pace by 20 bpm, or adding 2-pound hand weights. However, loading weight at the torso is of limited use, as it is highly impractical. Dynamic non-weighted arm activity is recommended as the most direct way to increase step training intensity via the upper body, while minimizing injury risk.

Chapter Five

Programming

There are a variety of class formats available for step training, ranging from classes of different levels (beginner to advanced) to combination classes mixing step training with traditional high- or low-impact aerobic dance. Depending on the chosen format, adjust your class design, movement patterns, and music.

Class Format

A typical, traditional step class includes:

Full-body warm-up (5–10 minutes)

Cardiovascular conditioning segment (20–40 minutes)

Post-aerobic cool-down (5 minutes)

Muscular strength and endurance segment (5–10 minutes)

Post-stretch (5–10 minutes)

Full-body Warm-up

This portion of class, which includes dynamic flexibility exercises, is essential, as it prepares the body for vigorous activity while providing an introduction to the types of movements that will be performed. Lead an active warm-up that incorporates movements both on and off the platform, using certain step patterns to reinforce terminology and movements. More complex movements might be taught at half-tempo, or taught on the floor as a low-impact routine while you perform on the platform to demonstrate the step movement. Additionally, consecutive stepping patterns should be executed at half-tempo if using faster music speeds beyond the accepted range of 118–128 bpm, which is common with beginning to intermediate classes that cannot warm-up adequately at a slower step bpm. All moves in the warm-up should be basic and low-impact to avoid injuries that can occur when cold muscles perform intense moves. Another important aspect to the step warm-up involves teaching participants about their space boundaries. A warm-up involving step moves allows participants to acclimate to the height and width of their platform, while dynamic floor moves provide information on the space available around the platform. A warm-up conducted entirely on the floor is inappropriate and ill-advised as it is not specific to the muscles used in step training, and participants then begin the step portion of the class without awareness of the platform dimensions.

Cardiovascular Conditioning Segment

This is the core of a step class, and should progress in both intensity and complexity from the warm-up and peak as the class level dictates. Intensity should be monitored either throughout this segment via the Ratings of Perceived Exertion method, with at least one heart rate measurement, or, ideally, by incorporating both methods.

Post-aerobic Cool-down

This phase of the class should run approximately 5 minutes, and involve similar movement strategies as employed in the warm-up. The goal of this section of the step class is to lower the heart rate to the appropriate level (below 110 bpm) to begin the next segment of the class. It usually includes standing static stretches, which lead into muscle conditioning work and then the final cool-down.

Muscle Strength and Endurance Segment

This might only include torso and mid-upper back strengthening work, which is highly appropriate. If additional strength work is possible, you should avoid working muscle groups fatigued from the step movements themselves (i.e., hip flexors, quadriceps).

Post-stretch

Lead the class through the stretching of all lower-body muscle groups, including the quadriceps, hamstrings, gastrocnemius and soleus, hip flexors, gluteals, and abductors.

Alternative Formats

The versatility of step training is a large factor in its success. There are a variety of step class formats available. In addition, the platform can be used as a prop in other class formats.

Step Circuit

In a step-circuit class, a variety of work stations are alternated to include cardiorespiratory and/or strength activities using the step. For example, one station might include traditional basic step patterns while the next might be a strength segment of

squats with one leg on the platform while performing lateral rais-
es with dumbbells. The choice of strength exercises is critical in
these classes, as the head must remain elevated above the heart
for cardiac safety and the leg musculature must keep moving to
avoid blood pooling in the lower extremities.

Step Interval

Interval training is an advanced performance-enhancement
technique that involves intermittent exercise of high intensity
followed by less intense recovery intervals where the frequency,
intensity, and duration of the intervals are fixed according to specific program goals. In a group exercise class setting where training is for conditioning rather than performance, step interval is
referred to as interval conditioning. It involves the use of step
training movements that alternate between steady state aerobic
work (via basic step maneuvers) and high-intensity anaerobic
work (via power moves). Interval ratios might be designed as
1:1, 1:2, or 1:3, where a set number of minutes of effort are followed with an equal, double, or triple number of recovery minutes
to complete several cycles throughout the class. Generally, the
higher the intensity level of the one-minute anaerobic work, the
longer the aerobic recovery period.

Combination Classes

A plethora of options are available under this heading, in
which step training is combined with another type of aerobic
activity such as high-impact, low-impact, or slide training.
Classes are usually designed to be half step training and half
an alternate modality. However, the format can also be pat-
terned after an interval class where a set number of minutes
are spent stepping followed by the other activity in repeated
cycles. The step circuit class is similar, with the alternate activ-

ity being strength work.

Muscle Conditioning

The step makes a wonderful prop in strength and conditioning classes, adding to the options available for working any muscle group. For example, squats can be performed with one leg on the step platform, which varies the actions of the leg muscles. Participants can sit or lie upon the step to perform exercises such as seated overhead presses with dumbbells or supine chest flies. The platform can also be held lengthwise, resting one end on the floor to aid in balance for activities like standing hamstring work. Finally, depending on the type of step equipment available, the platform can be adjusted to create an incline for variations in abdominal, chest, and leg work.

Choreographic Considerations

Most of the movement patterns in step training are 4-count or 8-count moves, allowing for easy choreography design. Beginner level classes should include basic movements that maintain 4- or 8-count designs. Movements that do not flow with most aerobic music, which uses 8-count measures, require significantly more planning and design. For example, a 2-Knee Repeater is a 6-count movement pattern. Movements at odds with the strong beats that accompany the 8-count measures of aerobic music can be difficult for some participants to perform, as they may not understand that a movement feels odd because they are moving against the natural beat of the music. Complex moves are more appropriate for intermediate and advanced participants.

There are certain movements possible in step training that do not follow ACE Guidelines for biomechanical and musculoskeletal safety. These include stepping forward off the front of the platform, performing movements where the platform is not in clear view, and some turning or pivoting movements. These moves are dangerous, and therefore inappropriate for almost all class participants in almost all situations.

Keep the platform in view at all times, directly or in the peripheral vision. Movement forward off the platform places the platform behind the participant, out of view. In addition to this risky position that requires a potentially dangerous movement to get the platform back in view for continued stepping, the act of moving forward off the platform can be biomechanically unsafe. Choreography that requires participants to step forward with their back to the platform can increase the vertical impact forces by as much as 25%, compromising the knee joint (Francis et al., 1991). Some instructors perform this move thinking it is acceptable for advanced participants or in the warm-up/cool-down portions of class when music is slower. This practice is not recommended, and you are advised against the use of forward stepping off the platform.

Other movements that place the platform in unclear view include grapevines toward the back wall (with the platform behind the participant) and Hop Turns away from the platform. Any movement patterns that leave participants at an awkward, indirect approach to the platform should be used minimally, and only with advanced participants. Use your judgment of participants' capabilities and skill level with each and every class, and design choreography accordingly.

Power moves include hops, runs, leaps, and jumps on the platform. In most instances these moves provide a high-intensity option for participants seeking a more vigorous workout. Power moves such as Hop Turns involve shifting the body weight while in mid-air. It is critical that you instruct against shifting body weight while either leg is weightbearing on the platform as this creates extreme torque on the knee joint (Copeland, Francis, Francis, & Miller, 1992). Provide alternatives to such moves in all cases. For example, walking around the platform for 4 counts is an option for participants that do not want to complete a Hop Turn. Choreography must be designed so that participants performing either option remain on the same lead leg to smoothly continue the step routine.

The Reverse Turn, a Turn Step facing away from the platform when on top mid-turn, is a movement instructors have included in their choreography as an advanced skill. Research is needed to clarify the safety of Reverse Turns. Current knowledge of knee kinematics during step training, based on research conducted in 1998 (Hoose et al.), points to possible extreme torque at the knee joint during this movement pattern. These moves should be limited and used only for advanced participants. A regular Turn Step is the biomechanically safe option to a Reverse Turn in choreography design.

You are responsible for the safety of all participants in class, and must design choreography appropriate to the needs and abilities of the class. An additional responsibility is to educate participants. More advanced participants have a tendency to partake of options they feel increase intensity and/or creativity, with or without a cue from the instructor. An example of this might include a Knee Repeater option where the third knee lift pivots backwards away from the platform, so that counts 7 and 8 of the movement require returning the body to the front approach position. While such movements may increase the complexity of the class, they usually force the body to perform movements that go against the principles of biomechanical safety for step training. Educate participants performing such movements, either during class or one-on-one, as to why these movements are not advised and the likely injury outcomes of regular use of these movement patterns.

Patterns that require a significant number of consecutive turning moves should also be used conservatively and only with advanced participants. For example, a Hop Turn into a Straddle followed by another Hop Turn requires considerable skill at shifting body weight. Participants can easily become disoriented with such movements, and caution is advised.

Music

Music Speed and Biomechanical Issues

One of the most controversial issues in step training is music speed. The original bpm recommendation from Reebok University regarding step training classes was 118–122 (Francis et al., 1991). After considerable research, these are still recommended as the most safe and effective cadences for use in the average step class. Research done in 1996 revealed biomechanically safe step speeds of 122–128 bpm for intermediate and advanced step exercisers, while showing that biomechanical safety is compromised at speeds above 128 bpm (Scharff-Olson et al., 1996). Despite these findings, many group fitness instructors choose to teach step training classes at speeds well above the recommended maximum. Although exercise participants might desire faster-paced music as they become more highly skilled and fit steppers, it is your responsibility to provide a safe class.

> You should analyze the participant make-up of each class to determine the optimal step speed between 118–128 bpm. For beginning level classes music speeds should remain within 118–122 bpm. Consult Table 2 for a complete listing of guidelines on step music speed for different class levels.

Take notice of participants' heights, as tall people with longer limbs cannot mechanically move as quickly as those with shorter limbs. Regardless of your height, if a class consists of mostly taller people the music pace might need to be a bit slower. It is critical that you watch the participants throughout a step class to make sure everyone can safely complete all movements within their range of motion. Music that is too fast will cause participants to have improper body alignment, leaning too far forward to generate the needed momentum to move up and down, placing stress on the lower back. "Groucho" stepping is a common occurrence when participants are forced to step at inappropriately high cadences, where slouching takes place because there is not enough time to step up to full extension during movement patterns (Figure 32). Additionally, participants stepping too fast tend to step too far back from the platform to maintain the needed forward lean to get back up on top of the platform quickly. Potential Achilles' problems arise because fast-steppers often have improper foot placement both onto the step (allowing the heel to hang off the platform edge) and off the step (bouncing) because there is not enough time to completely place the heel on the platform or floor to get the needed full range of motion. Fast music

Figure 32
Playing music
too fast results
in poor form.

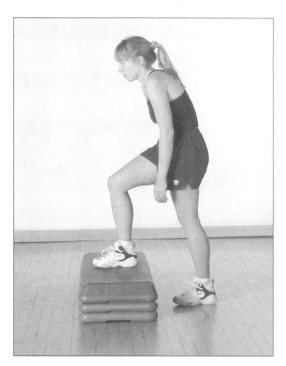

speeds can alter an individual's ability to perform step moves correctly with full range of motion, resulting in alignment variations that often lead to injury.

Consider music speed during the warm-up phase of a step training class. Typically, warm-up music speed is paced between 130 and 140 bpm to ensure an adequate warming of the core temperature and limb muscles. As these speeds are above the recommended step speeds, movements on the platform should be used minimally if warming up with music in this range. Methods for safety include incorporating a few step movements into the warm-up along with mostly non-platform movements and performing consecutive step moves at half tempo. Music speeds of 126–128 bpm, reserved for intermediate and advanced steppers, elicit the warming responses desired in this class segment. Warm-ups in this range of bpm should include less complex skills with some non-platform choreography.

Types of Step Music

There are a variety of national music organizations that provide step training music tapes or compact disks at appropriate beats per minute. ACE recommends that music be obtained from companies authorized to produce music according to federal copyright and licensing statutes. Since step movements most often occur in 4- and 8-count increments, purchase music that is blended by 8-count measures.

When selecting music, consider the audience and what type of music is most likely to motivate them. While advanced college-aged participants might enjoy top-forties hits, seniors would probably prefer big-band, oldies hits, or instrumental step music. Soliciting participant feedback and input are ways to ensure their needs are being met, and they appreciate the opportunity to provide input. Be sure to provide a wide variety of music to enhance participant enjoyment and continued interest.

Music Volume

OSHA (Occupational Safety and Health Administration) allows music volume levels of 90 decibels in a fitness classroom (ACE, 2000). Audiologists, however, recommend keeping music volume at or below 80–85 decibels, and using more base and less treble to minimize risk of injury to the hearing apparatus for both instructors and participants. Consider the audience when setting music volume. For example, seniors usually prefer a lower music volume. The teaching environment must also be taken into account when determining music volume as lack of a microphone, a large room, and poor acoustics all affect the participants' ability to hear cues and might necessitate decreased music volume.

Index

A

A step, 20-21
abduction repeater, 27
abductors, 69
Achilles' notch, 60
Achilles' tendonitis, 58, 75
across the top (lateral), 32-33
adaptability, 6-8
advanced level, 8
aerobic dance, 3
aerobic stepping. *see* step training
alignment cues, 53
alternate lead, 14, 17-18
alternate straddle down, 31
alternate straddle up, 32
alternating lift steps, 25-26
alternative formats, 69-71
American College of Sports
     Medicine (ACSM), 5
ankle weights, 63, 66
articular cartilage, 46
astride, 11, 13

B

basic step, 14, 15
beginner level, 8
bench aerobics. *see* step training
biomechanics, 55-61, 63, 65, 74
blood pooling, 70
body weight, role in amount of
     calories expended, 6
bouncing, 58, 59, 75

C

cadence, 7
calories expended, and
     body weight, 6
cardiac rehabilitation, 2
cardiorespiratory training, 4-5
cardiovascular conditioning
     segment, 67, 68-69
chondromalacia, 58
choreographic terminology, 9-43
choreography considerations,
     71-74
circuit training, 4
class formats, 67-69
alternative, 69-71
combination classes, 70-71
combinations, 15
cool-down, 67, 69
corner to corner, 22
cueing, 53-55

D

dangerous moves, 72
Deivert, R., 63
directional approach, 10-13
down steps, 14

E

environment, 61-62
equipment, 51-52, 61

F

fatigue, 45, 62
fitness level, 62
foot alignment, 44-48
footwear, 48, 60
Francis, P., 6
from the corner, 11, 12
from the end, 11, 13
from the front, 10
from the side, 10, 11
from the top, 11, 12
full-body lean, 46, 47, 50
full-body warm-up, 67, 68

G

gastrocnemius, 69
gluteals, 69
grapevines, 72
"Groucho" stepping, 75

H

half-tempo, 68
hamstring curl, 24
hamstring repeater, 26
hamstrings, 69
hand weights, 63-66
Harvard Step Test, 2
health limitations, 62
heart rate measurement, 69
hip flexors, 69
Hoose, R., 56
hop turns (pop turns),
    42-43, 72, 73

I

injury prevention, 55-61, 62, 72, 73
intensity monitoring, 51, 55, 68
intermediate level, 8
interval ratios, 70

interval training, 4, 70

K

Kasch, Fred, 2
kick, 24, 26
kick repeater, 26
kinesiology, 44-49
knee compression forces, 46
knee flexion, 56, 57
knee kinematics, 73
knee lift, 24, 26, 34, 35
knee rehabilitation, 2
knee repeater, 26, 27
Kravitz, L., 63, 64, 65

L

L step, 34-35
lateral (across the top), 32-33
lean, full-body, 46, 47, 50
left basic, 15
left turn, 30
leg abduction, 24, 26
leg curl, 26
levels, of participation, 7, 8
lift step
    alternating, 25-26
    repeater, 26, 45
    single lead, 23-24
    traveling, 25
lunges, 6, 40-42, 45, 60

M

metabolic cost of exercise, 2
METS (metabolic equivalents),
    4, 6
mirroring, 61
mirrors, 61
modifications, 51, 63-66
mood enhancement, 8

motivational cues, 53
movement cues, 53
muscle involvement, 48-49
muscular conditioning, 4, 71
muscular strength and
endurance segment, 67, 69
music, 74-77
music speed
and biomechanical issues,
74-77
for different participant
levels, 7, 8
warm-up, 76

N

O

P

Q

R

S

single lead movements, 14, 45
soleus, 69
space boundaries, 68
spinal alignment,
    46-47, 50, 53, 75
sports medicine rehabilitation, 2
squats, 42, 71
stability, 45
Stanforth, D., 5
static stretches, 69
step circuit, 69-70
step interval, 70
step orientation, 9
step patterns, 6, 15-43
step rate, 6, 75
step-test protocols, 2
step training
    adaptability, 6-8
    benefits, 4-8
    defined, 1
    energy expenditure, 4, 5, 6
    growth, 3-4
    history, 2-3
    low-impact nature, 1, 2, 3
    and mood enhancement, 8
step types, 14-15
straddle down, 30-31
straddle up, 31-32
stretch, 67, 69
supination, 48
supine chest flies, 71

T

T step, 34-38
tap down, 16-17
tap up, 17
teaching a step class, 50-66
    biomechanics, 55-61
    cueing, 53-55
    equipment, 51-52
    injury prevention, 55-61
    intensity monitoring, 51, 55

verbal introduction, 51
terminology, 9-43, 54
3-Minute Step Test, 2
torso weights, 66
traveling lift step, 25
traveling tap down. *see* turn step
travel step. *see* turn step
turn step, 28-30, 73
2-knee repeater, 71

U

up steps, 14
up tap/down tap, 18
U turn, 39-40

V

V step, 16
variations, 14
ventilation, 61
verbal introduction, 51
vertical impact forces,
    44-45, 58, 60
vigor, 8
visual cues, 55
voice inflection, 54
volume, of music, 77

W

warm-up, 67, 68
weight management, 5-6
weights, 63-66
whole-body lean. *see* full-body
    lean
Williford, H., 5
Woodby-Brown, S., 4
W step, 35

References & Suggested Reading

American College of Sports Medicine. (1995). *Guidelines for exercise testing and prescription* (5th ed.). Philadelphia, Penn.: Williams & Wilkins.

American Council on Exercise. (2000). *Group Fitness Instructor Manual.* San Diego: American Council on Exercise.

Calarco, L., Otto, R.M., Wygand, J., Yoke, M., & D'Zamko, F. (1991). The metabolic cost of six common movement patterns of bench step aerobic dance (Abstract). *Medicine & Science in Sports & Exercise,* 23(S140).

Darby, L., Browder, K., & Reeves, B. (1995). The effects of cadence, impact, and step on physiological responses to aerobic dance exercise. *Research Quarterly for Exercise and Sport,* 66, 231–238.

Francis, L. (1992). Step aerobics. *ACSM certified news,* 2, 1–4.

Francis, L. (1993). Teaching step training. *The Journal of Physical Education, Recreation and Dance,* 64, 25–30.

Francis, L., Francis, P., & Miller, G. (1991). *Introduction to Step Reebok.* Boston, Reebok International, Ltd.

Francis, L., Francis, P., & Welshons-Smith, K. (1985). Aerobic dance injuries: a survey of instructors. *The Physician and Sportsmedicine,* 13, 105–111.

Francis, P., Buono, M., & Francis, L. (1990). *The science of step training.* Paper presented at the 1990 International IDEA convention.

Francis, P., Poliner, J., Buono, M., & Francis, L. (1992). Effects of choreography, step height, fatigue and gender on metabolic cost of step training (Abstract). *Medicine & Science in Sports & Exercise,* 23 (S839).

Goodfellow, J., Hungerford, D., & Woods, C. (1976). Patello-femoral joint mechanics and pathology: 2. chondromalacia patellae. *Journal of Bone and Joint Surgery,* 58-B, 291–299.

Goss, F., Robertson, R., Spina, R., Auble, T., Cassinelli, D., Silberman, R., Galbreath, R., & Metz, K. (1989). Energy cost of bench stepping and pumping light handweights in trained subjects. *Research Quarterly for Exercise and Sport,* 60, 369–372.

Hoose, R., Lehnhard, R., Dewhurst, T., Pratt, P., & Hoose, K. (1998). Kinematic analysis of knee flexion during aerobic bench stepping and its clinical relevance. *Clinical Kinesiology,* 52, 52–57.

Howley, E. & Franks, B. (1997). *Health Fitness Instructor's Handbook*

(3rd ed.). Champaign, Ill.: Human Kinetics.

Igbanugo, V. & Gutin, B. (1978). The energy cost of aerobic dancing. *Research Quarterly,* 49, 309–316.

Johnson, B., Johnston, K., & Winnier, S. (1993). Bench-step ground reaction forces for two steps at three heights. *Medicine & Science in Sports & Exercise* (Abstract), 25 (S195).

Kennedy, M. & Newton, M. (1997). Effect of exercise intensity on mood in step aerobics. *The Journal of Sports Medicine and Physical Fitness,* 37, 200–204.

Koszuta, L. (1986). Low-impact aerobics: better than traditional aerobic dance. *The Physician and Sports Medicine,* 14, 156–161.

Kravitz, L., Cisar, C., Christensen, C., & Setterlund, S. (1993). The physiological effects of step training with and without handweights. *The Journal of Sports Medicine and Physical Fitness,* 33, 348–358.

Kravitz, L. & Deivert, R. (1992). Participant handout: the safe way to step. *IDEA Today,* March, 59.

Kravitz, L., Heyward, V., Stolarczyk, L., & Wilmerding, V. (1997). Does step exercise with handweights enhance training effects? *Journal of Strength and Conditioning Research,* 11, 194–199.

Kravitz, L., Wilmerding, V., Stolarczyk, L., & Heward, V. (1994). Physiological profile of step aerobics instructors. *Journal of Strength and Conditioning Research,* 8, 255–258.

La Forge, R. (1991). What the latest research has to say about step exercise. *IDEA Today,* September, 31–35.

Michaud, T., Rodriguez-Zayas, J., Armstrong, C., et al. (1993). Ground reaction forces in high impact and low impact aerobic dance. *The Journal of Sports Medicine and Physical Fitness,* 33, 359–366.

Reebok International, Ltd. (1996). Research says step Reebok bpm guidelines still safest. *Reebok Alliance News,* 9, 1–3.

Reilly, D. & Martens, M. (1972). Experimental analysis of quadricep muscle force and patellofemoral joint reaction force for various activities. *Acta Orthopedic Scandinavia,* 43, 16–37.

Requa, R., DeAvilla, L., & Garrick, J. (1993). Injuries in recreational adult fitness activities. *American Sports Medicine,* 21, 461–467.

Rupp, J., Johnson, B., Rupp, D., et. al. (1992). Bench step activity: effects of bench height and hand held weights (Abstract). *Medicine &*

Science in Sports & Exercise, 24(S12).

Scharff-Olson, M. & Miller, G. (1997). Stepping to a new beat. *Reebok Alliance News,* 14, 10–11.

Scharff-Olson, M. & Williford, H. (1996). The energy cost associated with selected step training exercise techniques. *Research Quarterly for Exercise and Sport,* 67, 465–468.

Scharff-Olson, M. & Williford, H. (1998). Step aerobics fulfills its promise. *ACSM's Health and Fitness Journal,* 2, 32–37.

Scharff-Olson, M., Williford, H., Blessing, D., & Brown, J. (1996). The physiological effects of bench/step exercise. *Sports Medicine,* 21, 164–175.

Scharff-Olson, M., Williford, H., Blessing, D., & Greathouse, R. (1991). The cardiovascular and metabolic effects of bench stepping exercise in females. *Medicine & Science in Sports & Exercise,* 23, 1311–1316.

Scharff-Olson, M., Williford, H., Blessing, D., Moses, R., & Wang, T. (1997). Vertical impact forces during bench-step aerobics: exercise rate and experience. *Perceptual and Motor Skills,* 84, 267–274.

Scharff-Olson, M., Williford, H., & Smith, F. (1992). The heart rate $\dot{V}0_2$ relationship of aerobic dance: a comparison of target heart rate methods. *The Journal of Sports Medicine and Physical Fitness,* 32, 372–377.

Stanforth, D., Stanforth, P., & Velasquez, K. (1993). Aerobic requirement of bench stepping. *International Journal of Sports Medicine,* 14, 129–133.

Stanforth, P. & Stanforth, D. (1996). The effect of adding external weight on the aerobic requirement of bench stepping. *Research Quarterly for Exercise and Sport,* 67, 469–472.

U.S. Department of Health and Human Services (1996). Physical Activity and Health: A Report of the Surgeon General Executive Summary.

Williford, H., Richards, M., Scharff-Olson, M., Brown, J., Blessing, D., & Duey, W. (1998). Bench stepping and running in women. *The Journal of Sports Medicine and Physical Fitness,* 38, 221–226.

Williford, H., Scharff-Olson, M., & Blessing, D. (1989). The physiological effects of aerobic dance: a review. *Sports Medicine,* 8, 335–345.

Woodby-Brown, S., Berg, K., & Latin, W. (1993). Oxygen cost of aerobic dance bench stepping at three heights. *Journal of Strength and Conditioning Research,* 7, 163–167.

NOTES

NOTES

NOTES

NOTES

NOTES

ABOUT THE AUTHOR

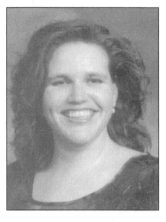

Sabra Bonelli, M.S., is the head of the Fitness Programs Department for the Mission Valley YMCA in San Diego, Calif. Bonelli received her master's degree in exercise physiology from San Diego State University. She has authored several *ACE Fit Facts* and articles in *ACE Certified News*. Bonelli is a member of ACE's Group Fitness Instructor Examination Committee.

Ace·
AMERICAN COUNCIL ON EXERCISE·
www.acefitness.org

YES, I would like to receive information on the following ACE certifications:

❏ Lifestyle & Weight Management Consultant   ❏ Personal Trainer
❏ Group Fitness Instructor   ❏ Clinical Exercise Specialist

Name _____

Address _____

City _____ State _____ ZIP _____

Home Phone (_____) _____

Work Phone (_____) _____

E-mail _____

Ace·
AMERICAN COUNCIL ON EXERCISE·
www.acefitness.org

YES, I would like to receive information on the following ACE certifications:

❏ Lifestyle & Weight Management Consultant   ❏ Personal Trainer
❏ Group Fitness Instructor   ❏ Clinical Exercise Specialist

Name _____

Address _____

City _____ State _____ ZIP _____

Home Phone (_____) _____

Work Phone (_____) _____

E-mail _____

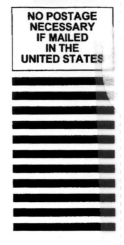

BUSINESS REPLY MAIL

FIRST-CLASS MAIL PERMIT NO. 22113 SAN DIEGO, CA

POSTAGE WILL BE PAID BY ADDRESSEE

**AMERICAN COUNCIL ON EXERCISE
PO BOX 910449
SAN DIEGO CA 92191-9961**

BUSINESS REPLY MAIL

FIRST-CLASS MAIL PERMIT NO. 22113 SAN DIEGO, CA

POSTAGE WILL BE PAID BY ADDRESSEE

**AMERICAN COUNCIL ON EXERCISE
PO BOX 910449
SAN DIEGO CA 92191-9961**